Welcome to your
new coeliac journey.

You've got this !!

Best wishes

Nicky x :")

About the author

Nicky Chilvers runs Gluten Free Little Cook and previously Nic's GF Bakes. She's mum to two teens, one of whom was diagnosed with Coeliac Disease in 2018 at the age of 9.

For anyone having a child diagnosed with this disease it's a shock to family life.

Nicky was determined her daughter wouldn't miss out going forward. She was left out once at school and that was enough.

She now helps other parents to understand how to manage family life & have as much normality in daily life as possible with practical steps and information to guide them in the right direction. Which is why she wrote this book.

Nicky is 51, a single parent and lives on the Herts/Beds border with her 2 teenagers.

To my two amazing, beautiful & intelligent
daughters. You are both incredible.
Your strength & support the past 3 years has
been second to none.
I love you both with all my heart.
*****

To my parents, sister, family & friends, far too
many to name individually here, thank you for
your love, support and encouragement that's
given me the belief I can do this.
*****

To the person who told me I was
'too capable' - thanks, I so totally am.
*****

And to Ted
Thank you for everything
xx

Contents

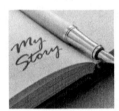

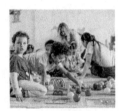

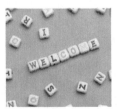

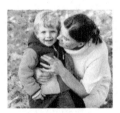

Sections

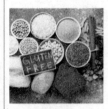

1 FIRST STEPS

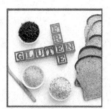

2 WHAT DOES GF MEAN?

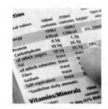

3 READING LABELS

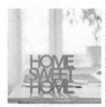

4 HOME LIFE & EATING OUT

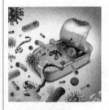

5 CROSS CONTAMINATION

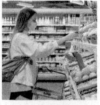

6 SHOPPING/ SNACKS/ TRIPS OUT

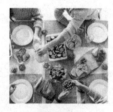

7 FOOD IDEAS

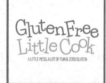

8 GFLC RECIPE FUN

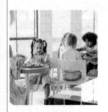

9 NURSERY & SCHOOL

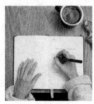

10 USEFUL INFO

Our Story

My daughter was 9 when diagnosed with Coeliac Disease following a blood test that was organised by the GP. It was a total shock

Grace had been ill on & off from around the age of 5yrs if not before.

She'd been a sicky baby, didn't like going to the toilet, didn't like sandwiches or bread but loved pancakes, pasta & homemade chicken broth.

She lived for pasta!! She often had a sore tummy, was lethargic, but nothing to say that it wasn't normal. It was just our daily life. But then she got really poorly and I was worried.

Ear infections kept coming, which caused her to be off school each September when they started. Pain, deafness, then sensitivity to noise. What 7-8yr old wears ear defenders to school? Something wasn't right.

Our Story

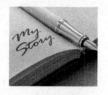

We cut out swimming lessons, kept water out of her ears and no amount of antibiotics touched it.

She turned a funny grey colour towards the end of 2017 and I really began to take notice. She looked really poorly, ghost like and the sore tummy's really caused her a lot of pain. Hot water bottles each night and nurofen.

But nothing was giving us a clear indication of what was wrong. Doctors said it was enlarged lymph glands from the ear infections, fighting a virus.... We were both at breaking point.

We took her to a private ENT specialist who couldn't find anything wrong. Keep water out of her ears.

In January 2018 I took her to the GP's again. I'm now really worried & request a blood test. The GP agreed especially as she was now drinking lots & really thirsty all of the time.

Our Story

I thought she had diabetes after searching the internet. She was grey, washed out, looked like death warmed up and definitely wasn't a well child.

The GP sent us off to the hospital & that Monday morning they took 7 vials of blood and tested for everything! Everything including glandular fever.

By Thursday afternoon I'd had a call from the surgery to make an appointment to discuss the results. With a 2 week wait. That just sucks as a parent. Panic mode kicks in.

Two weeks later I find out it's **Coeliac Disease**. Ergh, what? I had vague knowledge of it, but? The GP was very clear, **do not give up gluten**. I need to refer you to a consultant.

It could take months. At the time we were lucky to have private healthcare & she was seen on the 8th Feb 2018.

Our Story

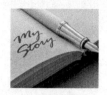

Grace was diagnosed by bloods alone as her TTG levels were high. That's how Coeliac Disease is diagnosed which is why you must continue to eat gluten.

128ttg on the first test, 238ttg on the second test by the consultant.

Since 8th February 2018, we've been gluten free & I've been immersed in the GF world one way or the other.

You learn to make the changes needed to keep them safe. To improve their health fast.

The smallest crumb of gluten could make them poorly, or using the wrong chopping board, a knife you've cut something with gluten in it.

It's scary and overwhelming, and quite draining in the first few weeks whilst you find your feet and get organised and clear on what you need to do.

GlutenFree
Little Cook

Our Story

I decided my daughter wouldn't miss out. On anything. And to date she has only been excluded once at school, and once was enough.

I wouldn't let it happen again.

Learning to bake gluten free is a test, you have to practice, learn from your mistakes, and there will be a few!! But practice & keep practicing. My first pizzas went into the bin along with the tins. But it gets easier.

But who am I to say what you should do?

I'm just a mum. But I am a mum to a coeliac child. I had to learn and thought there had to be an easier way. There wasn't anything that was specific to children when I looked, that could help me as a mum to a child who was poorly. No one understood, until I found other mums like me with a child the same.

Now I want to help you too.

GlutenFree
Little Cook

Our Story

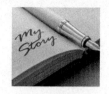

When your child is diagnosed, it's very lonely. You desperately need someone to understand, to connect with.

Friends & family whilst supportive, don't get the length you have to go to to keep your child safe & well. It's a total shock the length you have to go to & you need some reassurance that you're on the right track, something to refer to.

So I wrote this to help you.

If you can get your head around reading labels really well, cross contamination, having that back up snack in your bag, then you are going to do great.

Yes, there are other things to consider, school catering, birthday parties, family events etc, but that's for another day.

You have to start somewhere & that time is now.

Our Story

Yes, it's hard, there will be challenges, and your child will be left out on occasions despite your best efforts.

This book is about taking the first steps on your new way of life, getting going and feeling secure in everything you do going forward.

Once you've got everything in place, when you're used to reading labels on **EVERYTHING** that you ever buy, even if you buy it on a regular basis, it all becomes second nature.

You get used to preparing & serving their food first, not sharing bags of crisps or popcorn (win win at the cinema!), tipping not dipping crisps etc

But that's enough about us, lets get started. Take it a step at a time, go slowly, re-read, make notes. Don't get overwhelmed, I've got you & you can do this.

Nicky

GlutenFree
Little Cook

Child Record Sheet

CHILD'S NAME

DATE DIAGNOSED _____

TTG RESULTS _____

CONSULTANT NAME

CONTACT NUMBER _____

DIETITIAN _____

DIETITIAN NUMBER _____

CLINIC CONTACT
DETAILS _____

POST DIAGNOSIS BLOOD RESULTS

3 MONTHS	6 MONTHS
12 MONTHS	1.5 YEARS
2 YEARS	3 YEARS
4 YEARS	5 YEARS

Gluten Free
Little Cook

Welcome

Welcome to the Coeliac club!

Now, in fairness, it's not a club anyone would choose to join, but it's where we find ourselves as parents.

How are you doing? Overwhelmed? Lost? Scared & confused? Don't worry, grab a cup of tea, sit and let it sink in.

It is a huge shock. I was the same 4yrs ago. It's a surprise anyway, especially when you aren't expecting it. But it's your child. Your baby, and that is what hurts the most. If it were you it would be manageable, but I worried about all the things she'd miss out on.

But now you know, you can help your child get back to the best possible health after their Coeliac Disease diagnosis.

Their body needs to recover to get better.

Welcome

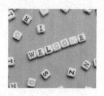

Maybe your child shows no symptoms so you never know if they eat gluten, or maybe your child, like mine, had terrible sore tummies. Nothing would soothe it.

As parents, we want our children to be safe, well & included. There are challenges to having a coeliac child. There will be lots of times you have to explain to them that they can't have what they want as its not suitable or safe. That can be heart breaking, but with planning & thinking ahead, some can be alleviated.

There are lots of things to understand & get your head around;
- what foods to buy
- how to cook & prepare food safely
- changing the food products in your house
- managing & minimising cross-contamination
- learning to read labels well
- being confident in keeping your child safe.
- plan ahead all the time

Welcome

- finding alternatives for their favourite foods
- helping them understand what is safe & what isn't.
- that their tastebuds will change, foods will taste differently for a whilst until you've tried them lots
- your freedom & flexibility will change in the early days - you can't just drop in at a restaurant & grab lunch
- finding 'safe places', venues that understand the cross contamination requirements
- always having a snack or back up packed lunch in your bag/car.

Amazingly, Coeliac Disease is the only disease cured by diet alone. Whilst it is lifelong, not cureable, it is treatable.

Let's get started.

SYMPTOMS

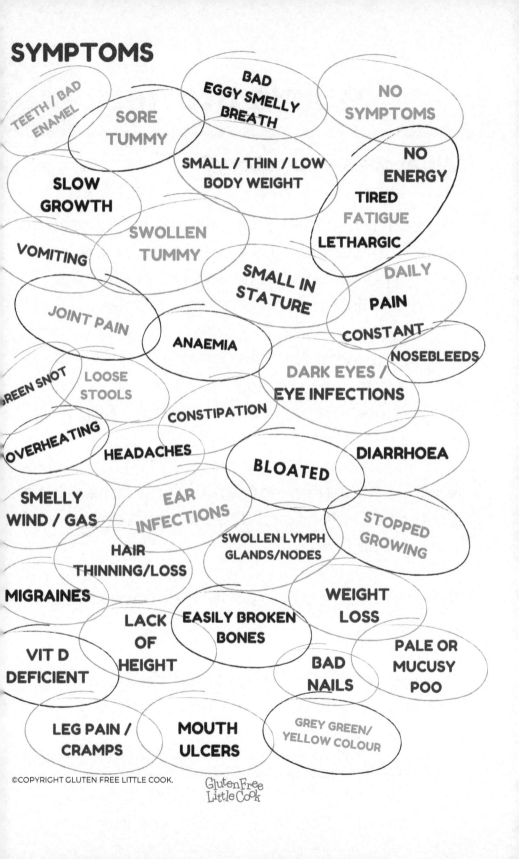

TEETH / BAD ENAMEL

SORE TUMMY

BAD EGGY SMELLY BREATH

NO SYMPTOMS

SMALL / THIN / LOW BODY WEIGHT

NO ENERGY

TIRED

FATIGUE

LETHARGIC

SLOW GROWTH

SWOLLEN TUMMY

VOMITING

SMALL IN STATURE

DAILY

PAIN

CONSTANT

JOINT PAIN

ANAEMIA

NOSEBLEEDS

GREEN SNOT

LOOSE STOOLS

DARK EYES / EYE INFECTIONS

CONSTIPATION

OVERHEATING

HEADACHES

DIARRHOEA

BLOATED

SMELLY WIND / GAS

EAR INFECTIONS

STOPPED GROWING

HAIR THINNING/LOSS

SWOLLEN LYMPH GLANDS/NODES

MIGRAINES

WEIGHT LOSS

LACK OF HEIGHT

EASILY BROKEN BONES

VIT D DEFICIENT

PALE OR MUCUSY POO

BAD NAILS

LEG PAIN / CRAMPS

MOUTH ULCERS

GREY GREEN/ YELLOW COLOUR

©COPYRIGHT GLUTEN FREE LITTLE COOK.

Gluten Free Little Cook

Mum's Stories

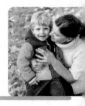

What was your story?

I asked mum's in a children's coeliac Facebook group what their children's symptoms were. The response was great and I compiled the symptom list and some of their stories.

Whilst the symptoms list on the previous page are not medically proven to be connected, it shows how diverse the reactions are & how it affects everyone differently.

No child had the exact same symptoms, which is why it's such a hard disease to diagnose, and can take so long.

Are your child's stories similar or have similar symptoms?

I believe that my GF teens ear infections were linked to the disease. She hasn't had one since being GF. Coincidence or ??

Mum's Stories

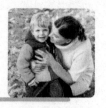

My 3.5yr daughter was tired all the time. It didn't make sense. My second daughter was 5 when diagnosed. She had a bad virus, couldn't stomach anything & the pain never went away so had her tested too.

My son's growth slowed right down at the age of 3. By 6yrs he'd gone from the 98th percentile to the 12th & was 10cm wide. He was very thin, pooed every 10 days & was tiny. No one would listen to me. A year on a GF diet & his feet have grown 3 sizes, he's taller, putting on weight & so much happier.

None. I had no idea she was coeliac until after testing. Once on the GF diet & healing, it became apparent she was smaller than she should have been. She was diagnosed after me.

My eldest always had stomach & water issues. Ear infections constantly. She was a sickly child & always in agony after birthday parties. We thought it was sugar.

GlutenFree
LittleCook

Mum's Stories

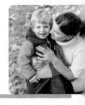

My son went from the 95th percentile to the 5th. At 3yrs, he's the weight of a 2yr old. We only noticed problems when he started nursery as everything at home is GF. Doctors aren't listening. I'm made out to be crazy, he's anaemic. I don't feel I'm being listened to.

My son is a different child since diagnosis. He had no energy before, was bloated, had constipation & anaemia. He was tested for other reasons but coeliac disease came back positive.

We were diagnosed at 18months. Sick 2-3 times a day, bloated, went down on the height & weight charts, pale, dark eyes. GP insisted it was a tummy bug for an entire year. Now she is a thriving 5yr old.

My daughter was 7 & had been ill since the age of 3. She'd migraines, throwing up & constant stomach aches along with bad wind & mouth ulcers. She's much better now.

Mum's Stories

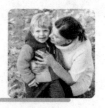

Our son was 4 but not growing. Smelly poos but not any of the typical symptoms.
I asked for him to be tested as his dad had been diagnosed the year before & my sister is coeliac too. He is now a happy healthy 9yr old who is definitely growing.

All these stories show that we've got something in common. That we aren't alone, that whilst we have children with the disease, it can show up differently in each & every child. Even adults

My child had earaches, sore tummies and eye infections. She didn't have a distended tummy, wasn't sick, and grew normally - I've overly tall children!!

There's one way to get your child better - a gluten free diet. It will be a challenge, they won't like the food in the first place. It will look and taste different. Their taste buds will need to adapt, get used to it, but they will improve.

Notes

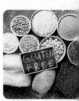

Section 1

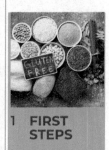

1 FIRST STEPS

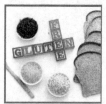

2 WHAT DOES GF MEAN?

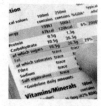

3 READING LABELS

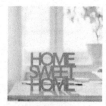

4 HOME LIFE & EATING OUT

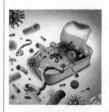

5 CROSS CONT-AMINATION

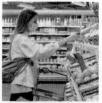

6 SHOPPING/ SNACKS/ TRIPS OUT

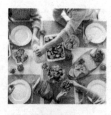

7 FOOD IDEAS

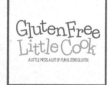

8 GFLC RECIPE FUN

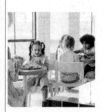

9 NURSERY & SCHOOL

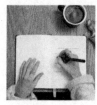

10 USEFUL INFO

First Steps

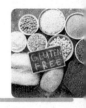

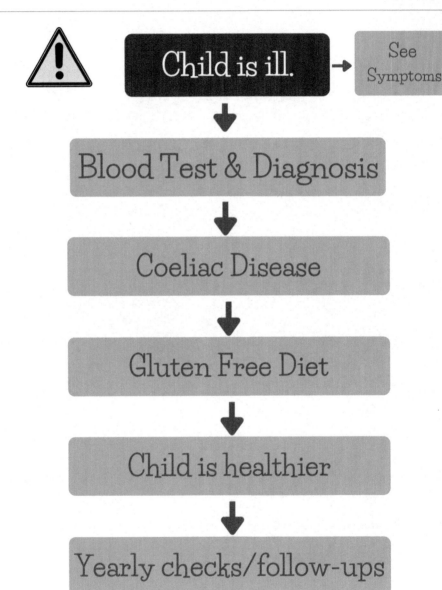

Child is ill. → See Symptoms

Blood Test & Diagnosis

Coeliac Disease

Gluten Free Diet

Child is healthier

Yearly checks/follow-ups

GlutenFree
Little Cook

First Steps

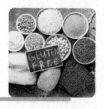

1   Ask the GP to arrange a full blood test including a Coeliac Disease blood test

2   Get results from the GP. Not a receptionist. Get a copy of the results

3   If positive - keep eating gluten.
GP should refer you to Consultant / Paediatrician

4   Keep eating gluten until the Consultant has completed additional blood tests &/or endoscopy & specifies you to go gluten free.

5   Confirmed - Go Gluten Free!!

GlutenFree
Little Cook

First Steps

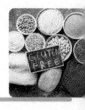

Getting Diagnosed

If your child is undergoing tests, please don't stop eating gluten

After the first positive blood test, you should be referred to a Consultant by your GP. They'll want to do their own blood tests to ensure it is positive before deciding on the next steps.

You need to keep gluten in your child's diet at this point. I know this will go against everything that you want to do. But it's necessary to avoid having to reintroduce gluten at a later date. Trust me, get diagnosed properly in the first place.

A blood test is the first & only accurate way to start testing for Coeliac Disease.

If you are advised to trial a gluten free diet by your GP - please don't - check with Coeliac UK in the first instance.

First Steps

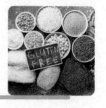

Getting Diagnosed

If blood tests aren't conclusive, your child may need an endoscopy. This is a procedure where they put a camera down their throat to look at their intestines whilst they are asleep under a general anaesthetic.

They'll be looking for damage to the lower intestines, to see if the villi are shrunken & any other damage that may have been caused.

Villi are tiny microscopic finger-like tentacles that filter & absorb the nutrients inside the intestines.

When your body thinks it's being attacked by gluten, it triggers an auto-immune response causing the villi to shrink into the intestine lining. This is why your child might not be gaining weight, look poorly or malnourished.

Their insides aren't working at their best.

First Steps

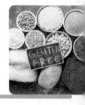

Diagnosis confirmed

You might be wondering what the test results say.

Results vary throughout the UK.

0-7 is what we were tested on yet some areas have their range 0-20, so ask what the 'normal' range is based on.

Above 7 is out of the normal range. Anything 10x above the normal reading is thought of as positively having Coeliac Disease.

Once your child is officially diagnosed by a consultant, all siblings should have the basic blood test including you as parents.

You child may be offered the gene test to see if they carry both markers for passing on the disease to any children. This is only done on those that are diagnosed as having coeliac disease.

First Steps

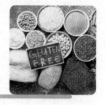

Diagnosis confirmed

It might be that the disease has been triggered by a virus or a food item that your child continually eats and/or that it is hereditary from you as parents. It might not trigger in you, but may trigger in your child.

Silent Coeliacs - those that have no symptoms or reactions at all. They have no idea that they have the disease.

The key thing to remember in the early days is that accidents happen. But you'll get the hang of it as you go, you'll find ways to work around it & manage day to day life & activities.

Coeliac Disease is an auto immune disease which is a lifelong condition that can only be 'cured' by a gluten free diet.

Gluten causes an auto immune reaction so that your body attacks itself internally.

First Steps

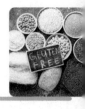

Diagnosis confirmed

It's important to remember that it's a lifelong condition. Any future blood tests will show levels dropping, and in future years when gluten is out of the system, it will show as '0' that you have any reaction or Coeliac Disease at all.

However, if you are not eating gluten, it won't show up in any blood tests. You or your child may even be told you don't have it any longer.

Remember it doesn't show up unless your child is eating gluten.

It doesn't mean its gone away. They'll always have it, their gut has simply healed & repaired.

If they're told 'you don't have it any longer', **they do**, it's just they're not eating gluten.

Stay on a gluten free diet excluding **Barley, Rye, Oats* Wheat & Spelt.**

Top Ten Tips

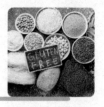

1	Coeliac Disease is a life long condition
2	It's an auto-immune disease not an allergy
3	Read the info given to you by the GP. Get a notebook for your notes
4	You'll need your little red book when you see the dietitian/coeliac clinic
5	Do your own research. Be aware that views & advice vary from country to country. Try to view UK based websites.
6	Look at joining Coeliac UK. The UK's leading charity for the disease.
7	Join Facebook groups for support. Remember you may get varying responses, and their advice may be incorrect or out of date.
8	Learn what you need to look for and how to read labels well and accurately.
9	Sort out your food cupboards at home.
10	Be prepared. Always carry a safe snack in your bag

Notes

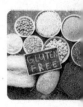

Where will you find help/support?

- **Coeliac UK website**
- **Facebook groups for children with CD**
- **Coeliac Bloggers on Instagram**

Notes

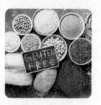

Section 2

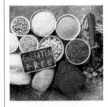

1 FIRST STEPS

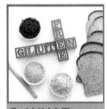

2 WHAT DOES GF MEAN?

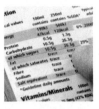

3 READING LABELS

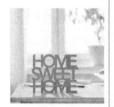

4 HOME LIFE & EATING OUT

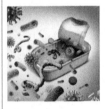

5 CROSS CONT-AMINATION

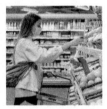

6 SHOPPING/ SNACKS/ TRIPS OUT

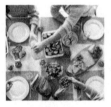

7 FOOD IDEAS

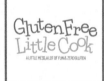

8 GFLC RECIPE FUN

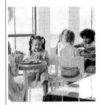

9 NURSERY & SCHOOL

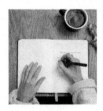

10 USEFUL INFO

What does GF mean?

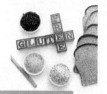

Going Gluten Free

But what does gluten free mean for you going forward?

Being diagnosed with Coeliac Disease means that your child has to cut out **all gluten containing foods & drink** from their diet.

Gluten is found in foods such as bread, cakes, pizzas & pasta. But as wheat/gluten is cheap, it is used as a filling ingredient in many other products.

Gluten is in **wheat, barley, rye & oats*** and is in foods you don't expect it to be in like ice cream, stock cubes, chocolate, sweets & supermarket own brand coca cola.

A handy acronym to help you remember what to avoid is <u>**BROWS**</u> - **barley, rye, oats*, wheat & spelt/semolina.**

What does GF mean?

BROWS / Gluten Free Oats

B Barley

R Rye

O Oats* - Oats must state they're gluten free to be safe. Regular oats are not suitable.

W Wheat

S Spelt / Semolina

What about oats?

Oats are naturally gluten free, but it's how they are grown and processed that matter.

They contain a protein called Avenin. This can cause difficulties in some coeliac's with the body thinking it is gluten as it's so similar. 7-10% of those with coeliac disease can't even tolerate gluten free oats.

What does GF mean?

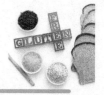

Gluten Free Oats

For a coeliac to have oats in their diet, it <u>must state on the packaging that they are gluten free</u>. Packets of gluten free oats are available in the Free From aisles in most supermarkets.

If you buy a product that contains oats, it must state that they use gluten free oats or that it's labelled a **gluten free item** which will then demonstrate gluten free oats are used & makes it suitable for a coeliac diet.

Some Consultants request you cut out oats from your diet for the first year & some don't.

When we were diagnosed in 2018 we were told by our Consultant that it was fine to keep them in our diet. That it was old advice to keep gluten free oats out of your diet for the first year and that it wasn't a problem. It makes it much easier.

Discuss your case with your Consultant.

Notes

Make some simple notes here to help you remember.

How will you remember about Oats?

What do you need to look for?

Notes

Section 3

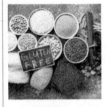

1 FIRST STEPS

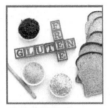

2 WHAT DOES GF MEAN?

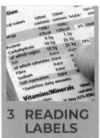

3 READING LABELS

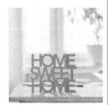

4 HOME LIFE & EATING OUT

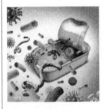

5 CROSS CONT-AMINATION

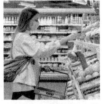

6 SHOPPING/ SNACKS/ TRIPS OUT

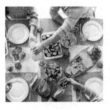

7 FOOD IDEAS

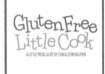

8 GFLC RECIPE FUN

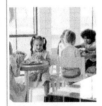

9 NURSERY & SCHOOL

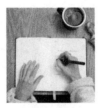

10 USEFUL INFO

Reading Labels

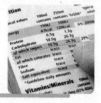

What to look for

Labels. If you can read a label, be confident you know what you are looking for, then you can shop quicker, save time and importantly save money.

Labels can be scary, you're not sure what you are looking for, big words etc. But you don't need to be frightened. A label has a job to tell you what is in the food.

The manufacturer has to tell you what is in a product. Gluten free is protected by law. But there are lots of products out there that are suitable, that aren't labelled GF as people, I mean 'muggles' aka normal people don't like seeing GF labels. They think of food as tasteless, crumbly etc.

It's a common misconception of GF food! Yes, there are some bad GF options out there, but, there are also some amazing ones too!

Reading Labels

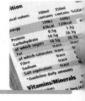

What to look for

Being able to read a label is key to ensuring your child is safe & that your wallet doesn't have a huge shock when you start food shopping.

Gluten Free food is expensive. Factories have to undergo rigorous processes when producing the GF foods and ingredients are more costly.

Knowing what you are looking for & how to minimise the cost as best you can is vital.

If you join Coeliac UK you get two apps to help you - **GF Food Checker** & **Gluten Free on the Move**. One scans food labels to show if suitable, the other helps you find restaurants/venues that are suitable when you are out & about.

Others to investigate are **Find Me Gluten Free, Glass Onion & Jolly Gut.** But remember to always ask questions & read labels. They don't always get it right.

Reading Labels

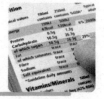

What to look for

But it is absolutely key that you know how to read labels too & don't rely on an app.

A scanning app is very handy in the beginning to give you confidence if you haven't read labels before.

But apps require updating on a regular basis & that doesn't always happen. They are updated at a later date.

There is nothing better than reading a label to ensure what ingredients it contains or whether there are processing statements such as 'may contain' making it unsuitable for someone with coeliac disease.

A label will always be up to date & override any scanning app or website.

Reading Labels

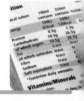

What to look for

Let's look at how to read a label.

- A label contains information about what's in a product
- The first ingredient stated is the biggest; the last is the smallest
- If an ingredient is made up of more than one component, they'll be listed in brackets after that specific ingredient
- If it states 'may contain' or 'contains gluten' it should be avoided
- If '**Barley, Rye, Oats*, Wheat** or **Spelt**' are highlighted in bold within the ingredients list, it should be avoided.
- If it states it's '**Gluten Free**' it will be safe as it is a legally binding term, protected by law
- If it states '**Gluten Free**' <u>AND </u>has **Wheat** or **Barley** highlighted too - <u>the Gluten free term applies. </u>They're highlighted for those that have additional allergies.

Reading Labels

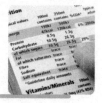

What to look for - Quiz Time

The main ingredient is **wheat**, then sugar, syrup & **barley** malt extract.

INGREDIENTS:
Whole Grain **Wheat** (82%), Sugar, Invert Sugar Syrup, **Barley** Malt Extract, Salt, Molasses, Vitamins and Minerals (Niacin, Iron, Pantothenic Acid, Folic Acid, Vitamin B6, Riboflavin), Natural Flavouring.
ALLERGY ADVICE: For allergens, including cereals containing gluten, see ingredients in **bold**.
May also contain **Nuts**.

Is it gluten free?

Yes or No

Toasted flakes of corn, fortified with vitamins and iron.

INGREDIENTS

Maize, Sugar, Salt, **Barley** Malt Extract, Iron, Niacin, Pantothenic Acid, Vitamin B6, Riboflavin, Thiamin, Folic Acid, Vitamin D, Vitamin B12.

Allergy Advice
For allergens, see ingredients in **bold**.

☑ Suitable for vegetarians

NUTRITION

The main ingredient is maize (corn) but then you come across **barley** malt extract.

Is it gluten free?

Yes or No

The main ingredient is **oat** flakes. It looks safe but what about the oats? What about may also contain?

INGREDIENTS
British Wholegrain **OAT** Flakes (34%), Fruit Pieces (Diced Cranberries (18%) (Sugar, Cranberries (6%), Sunflower Oil), Raisins (4%), Strawberry and Raspberry Flakes (0.5%) (Cornflour, Strawberry Puree, Raspberry Puree, Emulsifier (Sunflower Lecithin))), Glucose Syrup, Wholegrain **OAT** Flour, Sugar, Honey, Vegetable Oils (Rapeseed Oil, Palm Oil), Rice Flour, Natural Flavouring, Chopped **ALMONDS**.
ALLERGY ADVICE
For allergens, including cereals containing gluten, see ingredients in **BOLD**.
MAY ALSO CONTAIN: Other Gluten Sources, Other Nuts.
This product contains certified sustainable palm oil.

Is it gluten free?

Yes or No

ORIGINAL SALTED POTATO RINGS
Ingredients: Potato (Potato Starch & Dried Potato), Sunflower Oil (24%), Rice Flour, Maize Flour, Salt, Potassium Chloride.

May contain Milk, Gluten.

Hula Hoops. Ingredients look ok, but....what about may contain?

Is it gluten free?

Yes or No

Reading Labels

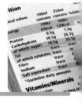

Getting it right

If you answered 'NO' to each of the questions for the labels, you are on the right track.

You need to apply this reasoning to **ALL** labels going forward especially if you are shopping in the 'regular aisles' & checking your home products.

- If it has one of the gluten items highlighted in bold, it's not suitable.
- If there are no gluten highlighted items in the ingredients of the product & no may contains, it should be suitable.

Neither Kelloggs or Walkers products are suitable in the UK. The risk of cross contamination is too high.

But, Walkers are known as Lays in Europe, and there, their crisps are stated as gluten free & suitable. As are the blue Doritos!! Grab a packet or two!!

Top Ten Tips

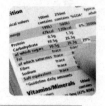

1 Reading labels is key.
Learn & know what you are looking for.

2 Look out for the highlighted ingredients - **Barley, Rye, Oats* & Wheat, Spelt**

3 Avoid 'may contain wheat/gluten', 'processed or produced in a factory that handles wheat/gluten', '

4 If it says gluten free on the label, it is.
It is a legally protected term in the UK

5 If it states it is 'gluten free' but has '**wheat**' listed, this is for those that have an additional wheat allergy. Same applies for **barley**.

6 The ingredients look fine (i.e. Hula Hoops) but they are a 'may contain gluten' so are unsuitable.

7 If there are no gluten listed ingredients, no possibility of cross contamination, it is suitable.

8 Gluten Free Beer - it is made with barley which will be highlighted. See #4 & #5

9 If in doubt, scan the item with a reputable scanner or on Coeliac UK.

10 And if you are really unsure, ask.

Notes

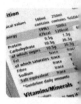

How will you remember to read labels?

What should you look for?

What's the acronym from S2 to help you remember?

Notes

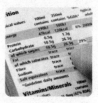

Section 4

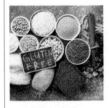

1 FIRST STEPS

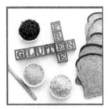

2 WHAT DOES GF MEAN?

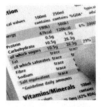

3 READING LABELS

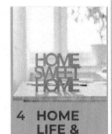

4 HOME LIFE & EATING OUT

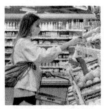

5 CROSS CONT-AMINATION

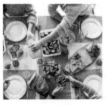

6 SHOPPING/ SNACKS/ TRIPS OUT

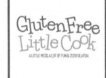

7 FOOD IDEAS

8 GFLC RECIPE FUN

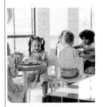

9 NURSERY & SCHOOL

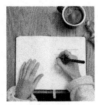

10 USEFUL INFO

LEARN TO READ LABELS WELL

Know what you are looking for - BROWS
Barley
Rye
Oats*
Wheat
Spelt

***Oats - must be labelled gluten free to be suitable for a coeliac**

STORE CUPBOARDS

- Check all ingredients
- Stock Cubes
- Packets
- Tins
- Flavoured Rice
- Worcestershire Sauce
- Soy Sauce

FRIDGE

Coeliacs need their own
- butter
- jams
- condiments / mustards

Get into the habit of using a spoon rather than a knife

FREEZER

Check all ingredients including frozen oven chips, everyday items you use that might have wheat/gluten.

Replace regular items with GF options.

Not everything in the Free From aisle is gluten free. Check the label

AVOID items from Kelloggs or Walkers as they're not suitable.

AVOID items that state 'may contain', 'may contain wheat' or 'processed in a factory that processes wheat'

TIP don't dip for crisp & sweet packets.

Diagnosed with Coeliac Disease?

What YOU need to know.

SCOOP with a clean spoon

CHECK your drinks. Often cheap cola has barley in it

TRY GF pastas etc. Find the one that tastes best for you

READ LABELS, save money. You don't need to shop for everything in the Free From aisle.

COOKING

- Cook GF items on their own trays
- Cook them at the top of the oven above gluten items
- Replace wooden items - spoons/breadboards
- Have a separate toaster or use toaster bags

CROSS-CONTAMINATION

A single crumb could make someone with coeliac disease ill.

- Keep your kitchen surface clear of debris
- Use clean pans/cutlery
- Silver foil is your friend
- Taste test dishes with a clean spoon each time
- Individual spoons for stirring

OTHER HELP

- Join Coeliac UK
- Download their food scanning app
- Learn to read labels
- Cook from scratch
- Find Facebook groups
- Instagram - search gluten free/coeliac

Home Life

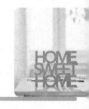

Time to make changes

Check your supplies. It's time to see what's in your cupboards and where the gluten is hiding. You'll be surprised!

You need to make some adjustments in your home to accommodate the new processes and procedures you need to put in place to keep your child safe.

A simple reorganisation of your kitchen, fridge, freezer & cupboards to begin with.

- Checking what you already have that can be used
- Find the items that are no longer suitable
- Know what alternatives you need to buy instead
- Find a way to separate what's GF

Let's break it down to some simple steps.

Home Life

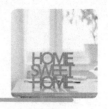

Time to make changes

Go through your food cupboards in the first instance.

- Check everything including stock cubes, packet mixes, curry jars, pastes, tinned items, soy sauce, condiments, mustards.
- Check the fridge contents - put a labelled plastic box into the fridge so that the coeliac child knows where their items are.
- Check the contents of the freezer & allocate a drawer/section to GF foods.
- Set aside a cupboard to put the safe gluten free items in. Then the gluten free child knows where their **safe place** is.
- Use freezer bags
- GF labels
- Sharpie pens

Remove items from use and replace with new if you can double dip into it i.e. get a knife in it. *See Cross Contamination section.*

Home Life

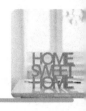

Kitchen Items

Toaster
You will need a separate toaster for GF items or use toaster bags to minimise the risk of cross contamination.

Saucepans/Frying Pans
Washed well (by hand & rinsed in clean water or by dishwasher) you will be fine.
Look to replace pans that are scratched or damaged.

I suggest you have a separate metal sieve/colander to drain gluten free items only such as pasta/vegetables.

Hob
Always ensure that you use a separate spoon for all saucepans. No double dipping or stirring two pans with the same spoon!!

Buy a few pairs of kitchen tongs. So handy when you don't want to touch food.

Home Life

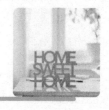

Kitchen Items

Oven

Give your oven a clean / wipe down.

Any gluten free food must now be cooked on a separate tray **at the top of the oven** to avoid cross contamination.

Cooking GF food at the top of the oven is so food isn't dripped onto or contaminated in anyway. Trays must be clean/well washed before use and/or lined with foil as required. Foil is now your new best friend!

Wooden Utensils

Wood can absorb gluten so it's believed, therefore you are best to replace your wooden spoons with either new ones for only gluten free use, and/or silicone ones.

In addition, you should replace chopping boards or better still have a designated chopping boards for your gluten free items.

Home Life

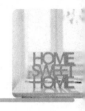

Kitchen Items
Fridge
Allocate a box in the fridge for the GF items & label it so everyone knows. Then everyone will know that they aren't to be used by others.

Your child will need their own butter & jams, anything that can be double dipped or get crumbs into. This is where squeezy bottles come in handy - honey, jam etc. Think of anything that could be double dipped & replace accordingly. Nutella is our main one in the house - my GF teen has her own. No one would want to share with her anyway! She can double dip to her hearts content!

Freezer
Ensure gluten free items are stored & labelled clearly. Allocate them a specific drawer, labelled bags or a box whatever works for you.

Check your frozen oven chips ingredients. Replace fish fingers with GF versions.

GlutenFree
Little Cook

Home Life

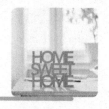

Baking / Cooking

Whilst checking everything, if you bake, you'll need to look at replacing the following due to cross contamination issues and anything that may contain gluten.

Most baking powders are GF but some aren't. Read labels & check

- Gluten Free Baking Powder
- Gluten Free Yeast - some quick brand yeasts contain wheat.
- Bicarbonate of Soda
- Xanthan Gum (this helps replace the 'gluten' to give elasticity)
- Gluten Free Plain Flour
- Gluten Free Self Raising Flour
- Cornflour

Most GF flours now are great to work with. Some cookbooks still refer you to make your own blend. I don't - who has time for that!

Gluten Free Little Cook

Home Life

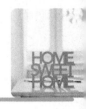

Checklist

CHECK EVERYTHING
- Check your store cupboards
  - ○ Baking items ☐
  - ○ Snacks ☐
  - ○ Crisps ☐
  - ○ Stock cubes/packet mixes ☐
  - ○ Soy Sauce/other ☐
  - ○ Pastas ☐
  - ○ Cereals ☐
  - ○ Mustard/Ketchup ☐
- Check your fridge
  - ○ Box to store own butter/jam ☐
  - ○ Label items ☐
- Check your freezer
  - ○ Create own space ☐
  - ○ Label items ☐

- Create a safe place for GF foods ☐

Swap gluten containing ingredients for safe Gluten Free options

Eating Out

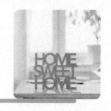

Restaurants & Takeaways

You're planning on eating out or having a takeaway with your child.

What venue is safe & how do you know?

It's a tricky one. You need to find venues near you that are suitable.

Coeliac UK have accredited restaurants & you can find them via the app & via their website. This means that they are aware of cross contamination & requirements of a gluten free diet.

There will be individual restaurants local to you that may be suitable. Check your local area, Facebook groups etc. But always double check they meet your needs & requirements.

Speak to them direct. Ask the vital questions.

Eating Out

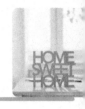

Restaurants & Takeaways

Asking vital questions is key if you want your child to be safe. If you get a good response which is clear & puts you at ease, fab. If not, avoid.

Questions to consider:
- Do you have a separate preparation area
- Do you use a clean pan/boiling water to cook the pasta (some places use a broiler & use the same water as for gluten pasta!)
- Do you have a separate chip fryer?

A good restaurant will:
- know to clean down
- have a safe clean preparation area
- minimise all risk of cross contamination
- put you at ease by answering your questions

Let's look options

Eating Out

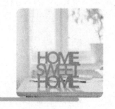

Restaurants & Takeaways

Fish & Chips

Yes, chips are potatoes & gluten free, but it's how & where they are cooked. A separate fryer is needed for them & any other foods that your child will eat at any restaurant.

Gluten isn't killed at high temperatures. If they say gluten is killed at high temperatures - leave & eat elsewhere.

They'll need to use separate utensils for the serving the GF items too. Watch how they serve & prepare their foods. If it makes you question yourself, don't risk it.

EG: if they use the chip fryer to cook the breaded gluten nuggets or battered fish, the the oil is contaminated so the chips will be too.

See if you have a good chip shop near you by looking in the *Gluten Free Fish and Chip shops in the UK on Facebook.*

Eating Out

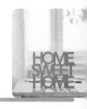

Restaurants & Takeaways

Chinese

It's the most difficult. They use wheat & soy sauce (contains wheat). It depends on their cross contamination issues.

There is an excellent Chinese restaurant in Manchester (Sweet Mandarin), and one in Cambridgeshire (Purple Diamond).

Look at Gluten Free Chinese takeaways and restaurants on Facebook.

Indian

Many Indian dishes are naturally gluten free, but you must check with each individual restaurant. Naan breads contain wheat but they use a lot of gram flour (chickpea) in dishes.

Pizza Hut

Accredited by Coeliac UK. A GF pizza is square & uncut. If in the restaurant they will bring you a salad from the kitchen rather than have you use the salad bar. Salad bars have cross contamination issues all over them.

GlutenFree
Little Cook

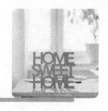

Restaurants & Takeaways

Prezzo

Accredited by Coeliac UK and my daughters favourite for a treat - especially their Fusilli & Spag Bol. We've had their takeaway & they have special GF labels to distinguish which dishes are GF foods & in a separate bag.
They only use fusilli pasta for GF options so you can determine it's safe.

Dominoes

Accredited by Coeliac UK. We've had no problems & it feels like a normal treat. Own separate section on the app. Pizzas are provided uncut to minimise contamination.

Pizza Express

Accredited by Coeliac UK. Great kids GF menu.
GF Dishes served on black plates. Dedicated GF pizza cutters when eating in. You can get dough balls/salad, pizza or pasta & usual puddings.

Notes

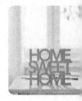

What questions would you ask to keep your child safe?

Safe prep areas?

General hygiene? Gloves, washing hands etc

Notes

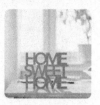

Section 5

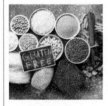

1 FIRST STEPS

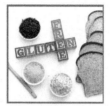

2 WHAT DOES GF MEAN?

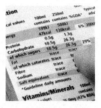

3 READING LABELS

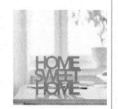

4 HOME LIFE & EATING OUT

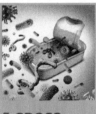

5 CROSS CONT-AMINATION

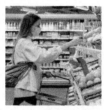

6 SHOPPING/ SNACKS/ TRIPS OUT

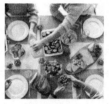

7 FOOD IDEAS

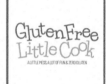

8 GFLC RECIPE FUN

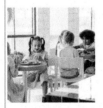

9 NURSERY & SCHOOL

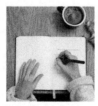

10 USEFUL INFO

Cross Contamination

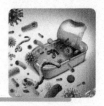

Let's talk Cross Contamination.

As mentioned in previous sections, Cross Contamination is probably the scariest side of Coeliac Disease. Just one crumb could make your child ill. Just one. Or the wrong knife in a jar, the wrong spoon stirring the wrong saucepan.

It's important to note that if they do accidently eat some gluten, known as being 'glutened' that their reactions may be stronger & more severe the longer that they are off gluten.

Before we go further, get a 'kit' ready so you can be prepared. Ensure that you have strawberry Nurofen, Calpol, Buscopan (age dependent). Maybe peppermints to ease their stomach as not many children like peppermint tea & ensure they drink lots of water to help flush out the system.

There isn't much else you can do other than cuddles and maybe a hot waterbottle.

GlutenFree
Little Cook

Cross Contamination

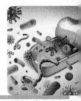

An example

Your child will need their own butter, jam, condiments etc. **Anything that could be double dipped is cause for contamination.**

For example, James makes himself a sandwich. He's not gluten free, so he grabs some butter, the cheese & regular bread. He butters the bread, crumbs go into the butter, he then cuts the cheese using the same knife. He puts his sandwich together, cuts it in half & puts the food all back.

Sam comes along.

He has got coeliac disease. He's gluten free. He wants a sandwich too. He gets **his** chopping board out, a **clean knife, his bread, his butter & cheese** from the fridge.

He makes himself a GF sandwich........

Cross Contamination

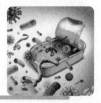

An example

The problem is that James <u>used</u> Sam's butter & cheese.

He used the same contaminated knife to butter the bread, to cut the cheese, contaminating them both. Crumbs in the butter & on the cheese.

Sam uses his safe foods believing they're ok. Sam eats his sandwich unaware that there's contamination & he is then ill. He's been glutened.

It takes just one crumb for most Coeliac's to get a reaction.

He was normally only sick pre diagnosis. Today, as he's been GF for 6mths, he is sick, has a sore tummy & diarrhoea. He takes anything from 24hrs to a week, to 3-4 weeks to get back to normal. It's important to minimise all possible risks & keep their items safe.

GlutenFree Little Cook

Cross Contamination

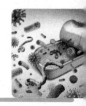

Make it clear

Ensure that all items for your coeliac child are labelled & in a container demonstrating that they are for them.

Even a large empty ice-cream tub will do. It doesn't need to be a new fancy box.

Write on it with a Sharpie - get them to decorate it with a few, put a sticker on it to show other family members that it's for the GF child only. Write on the products too so people can see. Write on EVERYTHING.

I buy different sized butter tubs to help distinguish what is for family vs GF teen which are then labelled or written on with a Sharpie pen.

I keep all GF items labelled plastic box (from Wilko) on the top shelf so everyone knows it's hers.

Cross Contamination

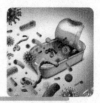

Top Tips

- Keep kitchen surfaces clean & free of debris.
- Allocate a kitchen area specifically for gluten containing items only
- Prepare gluten free foods in a separate area
- Have separate chopping boards for gluten free items / fruit / veg
- Use a clean spoon each time you try a dish you are cooking.
- No double dipping
- Always prepare gluten free foods first.
- Always serve the gluten free food first
- Invest in several pairs of kitchen tongs. They're fab for serving food items.
- Always have silver foil, kitchen roll, clingfilm
- Look at a separate toaster or invest in toaster bags from Home Bargains
- Crumbs = contamination. No sharing of bowls/foods/drinks.
- Tip don't dip is our house rule.

Cross Contamination

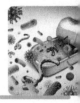

Top Tips

- Tip, don't dip - **sharing is no longer an option**. For example, James has finished his gluten sandwich, but dips his gluten covered hands into Sam's GF crisp packet without him knowing or sips his drink, uses his straw. Everything he has touched or drunk now has contaminated Sam's foods and drink.
- Buy squeezy bottles of ketchup, mayonnaise, honey, jams etc.
- Remember that gluten is not 'killed' at high temperatures. **Ever.**

And, one of our favourite things to help us remember is this; like Joey from Friends, Coeliac's don't share food!

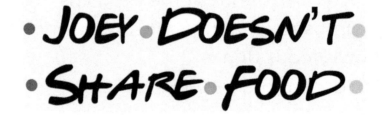

Cross Contamination

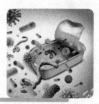

Buffets

Buffet's are sadly best avoided. Take a pre planned packed lunch for your child.

- The risk of cross contamination is too high.
- Other buffet grazers don't think when they are touching foods, picking it up & putting it down causing cross contamination.
- They touch sandwiches, then touch the fruit, the tomatoes, cucumber sticks, dive their hands into the crisps
- Using the serving tongs in one food bowl then another
- Making it all unsuitable for a coeliac
- If the person organising is aware of your needs, if they've catered for you, make sure they understand & check items are safe.
- If it is safe, then you are best to help your child at the very beginning & don't return.

Notes

How will you minimise cross contamination?

At home?

Out and about?

Notes

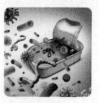

Section 6

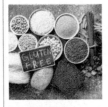

1 FIRST STEPS

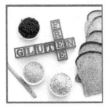

2 WHAT DOES GF MEAN?

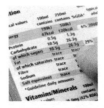

3 READING LABELS

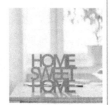

4 HOME LIFE & EATING OUT

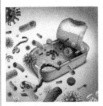

5 CROSS CONT-AMINATION

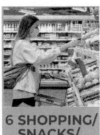

6 SHOPPING/ SNACKS/ TRIPS OUT

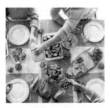

7 FOOD IDEAS

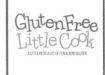

8 GFLC RECIPE FUN

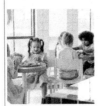

9 NURSERY & SCHOOL

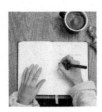

10 USEFUL INFO

Shopping

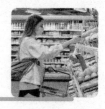

Get ready to shop

What to buy and where to shop.

Shopping is now more of a challenge. You will find your child tries lots of new things now, won't like them, but will like them in 6mths to a years time. Their taste buds need to adapt to the new tastes, textures etc. Be patient & give it time.

You'll find you now shop in more than one supermarket. They each bring something to the table.

Your food bills may be higher now. You'll need to shop in the Gluten Free/Free From aisles for your basic store cupboard items BUT not all the time as it will hit your waist and your pocket.

There are lots of items in the normal aisles that are gluten free, that aren't twice the price or twice the amount of sugar/fat/salt which is in a lot of processed GF foods.

Shopping

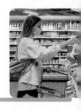

Get ready to shop

By reading labels well, you'll be able to reduce your costs.

*Note - if you use the Coeliac UK scanning app, Lidl and Aldi products don't scan. You've got to read labels. Neither have a specific gluten free section either. You have to look in the normal aisles & find what is suitable.

In regular supermarkets, in the Free From aisle you can pick up your gluten free dry goods such as:

- Breakfast Cereals
- Pasta
- Bread / Crackers
- Biscuits
- Snacks
- Cakes

If you don't bake, give it a go. It's cheaper, you know what is in them and they taste much better. See the recipe section from Gluten Free Little Cook that have made kids smile.

Shopping

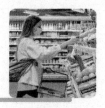

Get ready to shop

The rest of your shopping you should be able to do in the regular aisles; fruits/vegetables, some packet items, ready made sauces, ketchups, mustards etc.

Continue to read & check labels as you go, wheat/gluten hides in funny items. Mustard is one. Mustard itself is gluten free - in ready made versions they add wheat! Go for Colemans Mustard powder!

Fridge / Dairy aisles

- Yogurts are GF but check those that have additions to them - crunchie pieces etc.
- If you share a big family pot, pour it out or use a clean spoon to scoop it out. No double dipping!
- Own butters. Small spreadable tubs are great as they seal easily
- Petit filous, yogurt tubes
- mini cheeses
- Good calcium levels are important

Shopping

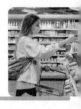

Get ready to shop

Meat

- Plain meats - whole joints, chickens, chicken breasts/thighs are generally GF
- You'll need to double check labels if it has a crumb coating/stuffing or gravy that it comes with it
- Spit roast chickens that are pre cooked in the supermarket are not suitable due to cross contamination
- GF chicken nuggets are in most supermarkets.

Sausages

- Most supermarket brands are GF fresh & some frozen
- You'll need to read the label to double check.
- Independent butchers some cater for gluten free. You need to check their processes match your needs.

Shopping

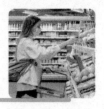

Get ready to shop

Fish

- Plain fish is naturally gluten free.
- If it has a coating or a sauce you need to check the ingredients.
- There are a range of GF fish fingers, fish pieces in the GF freezer section

Vegetables & Fruits

- All vegetables and fruits are naturally gluten free
- Wash and chop them on a suitable safe GF chopping board
- We've a chopping board designated for fruits/veg so that we know we are prepared safely
- If you buy pre-prepared vegetables, check the ingredients. Gluten can sometimes be declared on a label
- Potatoes, sweet potatoes, garlic, yams etc are all naturally gluten free

Shopping

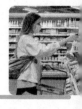

Get ready to shop

Pasta

- You'll try lots of pastas to see which one suits your child, they're not all the same
- Some have more corn/maize in them, others rice flour
- We tried lots before we found our favourites
- We now have gluten free pasta as standard as it's just easier when cooking family meals
- We like Sainsburys fusilli & penne pasta, Asda spaghetti, Barilla GF pasta from Tesco

Cooking GF pasta.

It's no different to regular pasta but I'd advise undercooking by 2m.

- To a pan of boiling water add plenty of salt
- Add the pasta
- Give it a good stir so it doesn't stick
- Bring back to a rolling boil 6-8m.
- Stir every so often to avoid clumping together.
- No need to add oil!! Totally pointless
- Cook to time/2m under & drain. Rinse.

Shopping

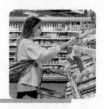

Get ready to shop

Rice

- Is naturally gluten free
- If it is a flavoured packet of rice - check the label.

Bread

This is a tricky one.

It's down to personal preference. Your child's taste buds need to adapt to the new textures & tastes & find something they like. Everyone is different. You can but test & try lots.

The ones we regularly buy are these:

- Warbutons Tiger Loaf gets good reviews as do their sandwich squares.
- Schar - their frozen rolls(6), their mini ciabatta (4) & hamburger buns (4) are great.

Warbutons square thins were also great when we first started.

Shopping

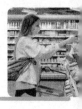

Store Cupboards
Check your store cupboards.

Tinned Goods
- Many tinned items are GF, tinned tomatoes, pulses, beans etc
- You'll need to check labels
- Handy tip - Heinz baked beans & pork sausages are GF!! A handy quick lunch
- Got packets of lentils? They will probably have a 'may contain' on them. However, you can wash them and they will be ok to use. Soak, wash and rinse well and they'll be ok to use.

I like to have the ingredients of my store cupboard all gluten free making it safe whenever I cook. I then don't have to worry or think twice when I grab the Soy Sauce or other condiments. I'm not second guessing myself. It's much easier!

Shopping

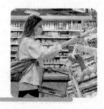

Simple swaps

Simple swaps are easy & no different to taste.

- Daddies Brown Sauce is swapped for Tesco brown sauce
- Soy Sauce - buy a GF version
- Marmite - Tesco or Sainsburys own brand is safe
- Worcestershire Sauce - swapped to a GF alternative
- Stock cubes - Kallo or other GF brand
- Bisto - buy the GF version
- Vinegar - Cider/Apple/Spirit vinegar
  - Barley Malt Vinegar (nor barley malt extract) are no longer recommended by Coeliac UK unless stated as GF. You can buy a GF Fish & Chip shop vinegar from Morrisons or your local chip shop

If you bake, you'll need GF flour going forward. And as before, to replace your baking supplies.

Shopping

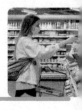

Store Cupboards

Breakfast

- Cereals need to be purchased from the Free From aisle
- Each supermarket has lots of varieties - mind the sugar content
- No 'own brand' supermarket cereal is deemed suitable any longer (they used to be classified as ok by Coeliac UK) but they are requiring changes from the manufacturers.
- Porridge - as in Section 2, anything with oats in it must state it uses GF oats
- Ready Brek is not GF & is not suitable. Try whizzing up some GF oats in a blender to get a similar consistency
- Other alternatives for oats if your child can't tolerate GF oats are rice flakes, quinoa flakes, millet flakes and amaranth
- Homemade GF pancakes or waffles. Cheap and easy to do with eggs, gf flour & milk.

Shopping

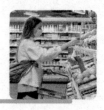

Snacks
Crisps
- There are lots of GF crisps in the normal aisle including Tesco/Sainsburys/Aldi /Asda own brands so your child won't miss out.
- Seabrooks are totally GF & have lots of flavours. Multi bags can often be bought in B&M/Home Bargains/Lidl/Morrisons
- Tesco prawn shells are GF, as are their bunny crisps, pom bears, cheese balls & multi pack crisps.
- Aldi & Lidl have GF crisps
- **Always double check & read the label**

Chocolate
Most chocolate is gluten free but there are some that are 'may contain'.
- No more Mars bars, Twix's, Maltesers or Kit Kats* or Smarties!
- Cadbury's have excellent labelling so check each bar. You can't eat the larger chocolate bars but you can eat their chocolate buttons.

Shopping

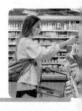

Snacks

- Galaxy bars are GF as are some bars in Aldi, and regular supermarkets
- Our top snacking list (the GF teen constantly snacks & loves) Flakes, Crunchies, Galaxy, Minstrels, Reese's (mind one of their new bars has pretzels in), Snickers, Twirls, Aero bars, Aero balls
- **Do always check the label.**

*Nestle Kit Kat have created small Easter Bunnies and Christmas Santa's (along with an advent calendar) that are GF.

The crispy pieces are made with rice flour & suitable for a coeliac. Definitely one to watch out for at Christmas and Easter. Stock up whilst you see them.

The regular Kit Kat's are still not suitable.

GlutenFree
Little Cook

Shopping

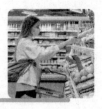

Snacks

Sweets

- Lots of sweets are GF but you need to check labels
- Party sweet cones should be avoided unless sweets remain in wrappers
- Strawberry laces often contain wheat
- Smarties contain wheat & are unsuitable
- Liquorice is one to watch out for as it contains wheat
- Remember tip, don't dip!

These are just some that are on our suitable list:

- Haribos
- Dib Dabs
- Moams
- Skittles
- Starbursts
- Kinder bars - *not buono ones
- Fudge
- Fruit-ellas
- Mentos

Shopping

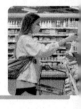

Snacks

Drinks

- Check all cordials/juices etc to ensure they don't contain wheat or barley.
- Fizzy drinks from dispensers are best avoided for possible contamination
- Bottles or cans are preferential
- Mind supermarket own brand colas - they often contain barley
- Don't share bottles of water

Alcohol

- My children use to have a Sunday treat of a weak shandy made by Grandpa. Obviously normal beer is no longer an option, but there are lots of GF beers available
- Wine is GF, and the majority of gins/vodkas are too. But some flavoured ones are not
- Baileys is GF and most if not all ciders are GF
- As always, check labels, check with the manufacturer

Shopping

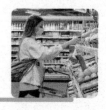

Treats & Trips Out

Cinema Popcorn
- Popcorn is generally GF at the movies - we've never had a problem
- Buy a large bag & decant it to cups you take with you or a paper bag from the pick n mix section
- Check their allergy list online. Be prepared, allergy sheets are a challenge at best
- Avoid the pick n mix sweets. Cross contamination risk is too high
- Avoid other foods/nachos etc
- Slushies - cherry/raspberry is ok

Ice Cream
- Always check the ingredients. Gluten can be used in cheaper ice cream.
- Lots of ice lollies are gluten free
- Avoid Nobbly Bobblys and the push up Rowntree Fruit Pastilles - they contain gluten.
- **Always read & check labels**

Gluten Free
Little Cook

Shopping

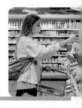

Treats & Trips Out

*Ice Cream Van.

- Buy safe items (lollies) that are pre wrapped
- Ice cream vans 'Mr Whippy' etc. Their ice cream is normally safe as its cream & sugar. Check with the vendor.
- Ask for a bowl/tub of ice cream
- Ensure the vendor doesn't touch the insides of the bowl (he may have handled wheat cones prior to this)

*We do buy ice cream from our local van. He now knows what we can't have. But we avoid the Flakes & provide our own.
Whilst Flakes are GF, my gf child was glutened due to handling (the vendor was handling cones, dipping his hand into the flakes, cross contamination). I believe that's what made her ill once when I was put on the spot with her wanting an ice cream like her friends, our first time attempting the ice cream van etc etc.
I wasn't prepared. It happens. So now we just have the ice cream!

Notes

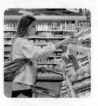

Notes

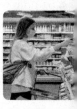

Section 7

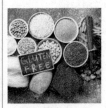

1 FIRST STEPS

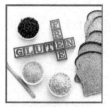

2 WHAT DOES GF MEAN?

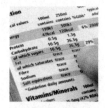

3 READING LABELS

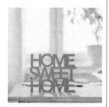

4 HOME LIFE & EATING OUT

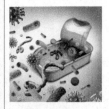

5 CROSS CONT-AMINATION

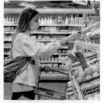

6 SHOPPING/ SNACKS/ TRIPS OUT

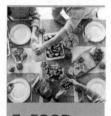

7 FOOD IDEAS

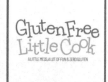

8 GFLC RECIPE FUN

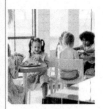

9 NURSERY & SCHOOL

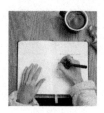

10 USEFUL INFO

Food Ideas

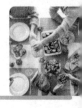

Everyday Foods / Alternatives

We've covered most food areas, but what about ideas for breakfasts, lunch boxes and dinners?

Here's a quick starter list. What else can you add?

Breakfast
- Smoothies - add avocado!
- Homemade breakfast gf oat bars
- Overnight gf oats
- Porridge
- Eggs - boiled, scrambled, poached
- Bacon
- Sausages & cooked tomatoes
- Beans on toast
- GF Pain au Chocolats (Schar)
- GF Toast
- GF Pancakes
- GF Waffles - see Becky Excell recipe online

Food Ideas

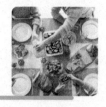

Lunch

LUNCHBOXES

- Make your own lunchables - roll up ham, fill with cheese etc.
- Mini Cheeses, Yogurts
- Hummus - carrot/cucumber sticks
- Apples & peanut butter*
- Raisins - *have cheese after to protect teeth*
- Veg/Fruit muffins, Pizza Pin Wheels
- Soup or spaghetti bolognese in a Thermos
- Dinosaur pasta (Morrisons) & veg/meats
- GF Sausage Rolls / GF Pizza
- GF Bread rolls / Wraps / Pitta breads with favourite fillings
- GF nuggets/Chicken goujons
- Mini sausages / Hotdogs / pepperoni
- Rice Cakes / Crackers / Crisps / Schar Pretzels / Popcorn
- Leftover dinner for lunch the next day

Food Ideas

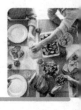

Dinner

- GF Spaghetti bolognese (GF pasta)
- GF Lasagne
- Chicken Curry & Rice
- GF Pizza
- Roast dinners - with GF yorkshire puddings
- Chicken nuggets & chips (check chips!)
- Homemade GF burgers & chips
- Homemade or bought GF pizzas
- Fish fingers
- Sausages
- Salmon & sweet potato wedges
- Garlic bread - make your own with pre bought gf baguettes.

Any of your normal day to day recipes that you'd cook, you just need to adapt them to a gluten free diet - it's not hard, just takes a little thinking on some occasions:

- Swap the wheat flour for GF flour
- Use cornflour to thicken dishes
- Use GF stock cubes
- Find ready made sauces that are GF

Ideas

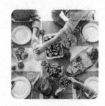

GF Foods & normal GF options

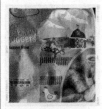
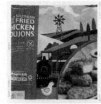
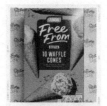
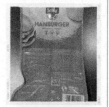

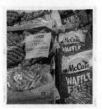
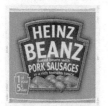
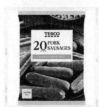
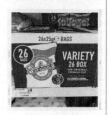

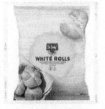
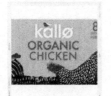
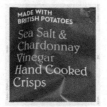
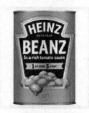

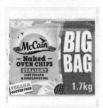
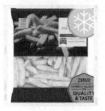
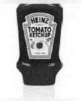
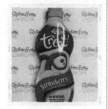

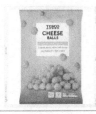
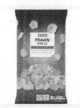
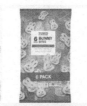
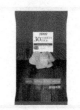

Gluten Free
Little Cook

Notes

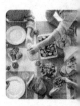

What meals does your child love?

How can you convert them to be gluten free?

What needs to change? Soy sauce?

Notes

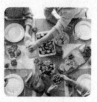

Section 8

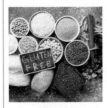

1 FIRST STEPS

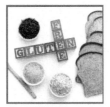

2 WHAT DOES GF MEAN?

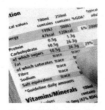

3 READING LABELS

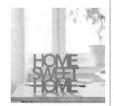

4 HOME LIFE & EATING OUT

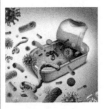

5 CROSS CONT-AMINATION

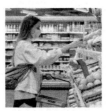

6 SHOPPING/ SNACKS/ TRIPS OUT

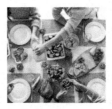

7 FOOD IDEAS

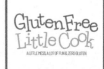

8 GFLC RECIPE FUN

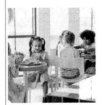

9 NURSERY & SCHOOL

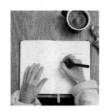

10 USEFUL INFO

Recipe Ideas

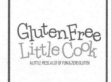

Gluten Free Little Cook

I had an idea one Saturday morning.

I was being bombarded by baking kits on Facebook. I'd obviously clicked on something to see what they offered. But no kits were suitable for us. We had gluten free requirements. So I wondered what was out there. Nothing specific for kids. So I set about sorting out something that could be easily done, created to be fun and make tasty treats.

Gluten Free Little Cook began.

It's developed over the past year, it puts smiles on faces and gives the children the choice on how to create their bakes. I can give them the idea and guidance, but they need to decide the outcome. If they want to eat the chocolate and not put it in the cake - who am I to decide what they do!

That is totally up to them!!

Gluten Free Little Cook Recipe - Lemon Drizzle

Equipment Required	Dry Ingredients *(supplied)*	Wet Ingredients *(not supplied)*
1 x large mixing bowl 3 x small bowl Mixing Spoons / Spatula Skewer or Cocktail Stick 1 x Tablespoon Mini foil tray or 1lb loaf tin Grater Knife & chopping board Pastry brush	85g GF SR Flour 85g Granulated Sugar	85g Butter* (plant or dairy) room temperature 2 eggs 1 Lemon (washed) (Optional – milk or lemon juice) Oil
	Icing 50g Granulated Sugar	Lemon juice from lemon above.

Note: *if you have an electric hand whisk or a food mixer, feel free to use it following the same steps. It helps make it super light & fluffy – or mix totally by hand. Either is fine.*

Method

Step 1	Heat oven to 160c Grease your mini foil tray/loaf tin or line your loaf tin with baking parchment.
Step 2	• Beat together your butter* and sugar together until pale and fluffy **Don't forget to check how fresh your egg is first! See how on your activity!** • Crack an egg into the small bowl. Check for any shell pieces & remove if there are any • Add one egg at a time to the mixture, mix well and repeat with the second egg. • Scrape down the sides of the bowl to ensure all the mixture is mixing together.
Step 3	• Next you need to make lemon zest. You make it by removing the skin of a lemon with a grater. The skin is known as the rind and by making lemon zest you are cutting the lemon skin into tiny pieces. And it smells super summery. • Have your grater on a chopping board or over your mixing bowl and rub your lemon over the smallest grater option to make zest. Ask mum or dad which is the best option. **MIND YOUR FINGERS. DO IT SLOWLY AND CAREFULLY until the lemon rind is gone** • You want to take off just the rind of the lemon until it shows white. The white is known as the pith & it doesn't taste too good. Add the zest to the mixing bowl. • Cut the lemon in half and squeeze the juice into one of the small bowls. You can use a fork inserted into the lemon flesh and twist it to help get the juice out. • Put the bowl to one side
Step 4	• Add the GF SR Flour to the mixing bowl. Mix it well until combined and no lumps. • If it is looking or feeling too thick, add 2 tablespoons of milk (plant or dairy) or for an extra lemon kick, add 2 tablespoons of your squeezed lemon juice. Save the rest of the lemon juice for now. Pour your mixture into your greased/lined tray or tin.
Step 5	• Place into a hot oven – be careful and ask a grown up to do this for you. • Bake for 20m. Test with a skewer to see if it comes out clean. Cook for a further 5m if not. Repeat. Once cooked, golden & skewer is clean, place on the side to cool.
Step 6	• Let the cake cool for 5m. Poke small holes gently all over the cake. • Add the small sugar packet to the lemon juice. Mix well. Spoon the lemon sugar mixture over the cake whilst warm to create a crisp coating as it cools.

Gluten Free Little Cook Recipe - Vanilla Cupcakes

Equipment Required	Dry Ingredients (supplied)	Wet Ingredients (not supplied)
1 x large mixing bowl 1 x small bowl Mixing Spoons / Spatula Skewer or Cocktail Stick Measuring spoons – tsp & tbsp 2 x teaspoons & 2 dessert spoons 1 cupcake baking tray & Wire Cake Rack Medium Ice-cream Scoop	110g GF SR Flour 110g Caster Sugar	110g *butter/dairy free block – room temp 2 eggs ½ tsp Vanilla Extract
	ICING Icing Sugar GF sprinkles	2-3 tbsp Boiled water Alternatives: Lemon Juice (optional) 100g butter (optional)

*Note: If you have an electric hand whisk or a food mixer, feel free to use it following the same steps.
I made these by hand just in case you don't.*

Method	
Step 1	Heat oven to 180c/160c Fan Pop your 12 cup cake cases into the tray ready for filling
Step 2	Beat together your *butter and caster sugar together until pale and fluffy. Crack an egg into the small bowl. Check for any shell pieces. Add an egg one at a time to the mixture until combined. Scrape down the sides of the bowl to ensure all the mixture is mixed together.
Step 3	Add the vanilla extract and the gluten free self raising flour Mix together until combined so there are no lumps & all combined.
Step 4	Put the mixture into the cases by using two dessert spoons (scoop with one and scrape with the other into the cupcake case) or use a small ice cream scoop. Try to keep them all the same size so they cook evenly.
Step 5	Place into your hot oven – be careful and ask a grown up to do this for you. Bake for 15 minutes until golden brown. Check they are cooked at 15m by inserting a skewer into the middle of the cakes. If it comes out clean, they are done. If it has cake mixture on it, they need a little longer. Give them an extra minute & try again.
Step 6	When cooked, place the tray on the side for 5 minutes. Carefully remove the cakes from the tin and put them onto a wire rack to cool.
Step 7	Place the icing sugar into a clean bowl, add 1-2 tbsps of hot water. Mix well. You are looking for a 'glue like consistency'. You may well need to add more water. You can add food colouring or use lemon juice instead of water for a tasty lemon icing. **Optional alternative** - If you wanted to make your cakes more fancy, you could add 100g soft butter and ½ vanilla extract to the icing sugar instead. Beat until smooth (a mixer helps!). Then spoon the buttercream icing onto the top of the cupcakes.
Step 8	When your cakes are fully cold, cover with icing using 2 teaspoons. Scoop some icing onto one spoon and scrape the icing off with the other spoon onto the cake. Shake or spoon your sprinkles onto the icing whilst its wet. Insert cupcake picks if made/using.

Gluten Free Little Cook Recipe - GF Oat Cookies

Equipment Required	Dry Ingredients (*supplied*)	Wet Ingredients (*not supplied*)
1 x large mixing bowl 1 x small plate 1-2 x small bowls Spatula 1 tablespoon 1 baking tray 1 fork 1 cup/warm water	100g GF Oats 50g Raisins 50g Chocolate / DF Chocolate Pinch of salt	1 ripe banana 2tbsp Vegetable oil 2 tbsp Honey Oil or baking paper for baking tray

Tie your hair back, wash your hands & pop on an apron.
Wipe down your kitchen cooking surface so it's clean and ready to go!

Method	
Step 1	Prepare your baking tray with a brush of oil or line it with baking paper
Step 2	• Peel your banana. • Place the banana onto a plate mash with a fork until nice and smooth. • Scrape the mashed banana into the large bowl
Step 3	• Add the gluten free oats, vegetable oil and 2 tablespoons of honey. • **Top Tip** – to make it easier to measure the honey, put your tablespoon into a cup of warm water first – then it will slide off more easily. Then scoop or pour the honey into your spoon from the jar or if you have squeezy honey, pour it into the spoon. (make sure the jar of honey is safe from cross contamination!) • Mix well • Leave it for 10 minutes covered with a tea towel. It helps the oats become moist.
Step 4	• Turn on your oven to heat to 170c • Add the chocolate and the raisins to the mixture in the mixing bowl • Stir well so the chocolate and raisins are evenly mixed
Step 5	• Half fill a small bowl with cool water • Wet the palms of your hands • Using a clean tablespoon, scoop out some mixture and gently shape it into a ball in the palms of your hands. • Place your cookie on your prepared tray. • Using a fork or your hands, flatten the cookie a little. • Repeat until you've used up all the mixture
Step 6	• Place your baking tray into the oven *Ask an adult for help • Cook for 15m • They'll go a light golden colour but not too dark.
Step 7	• Cool on the baking tray whilst they firm up.
Step 8	Then you get to choose to eat your cookies when warm or cold.

Gluten Free Little Cook Recipe - GF Rocky Road

Equipment Required	Dry Ingredients (*supplied*)	Wet Ingredients (*not supplied*)
1 x large mixing bowl & 1 x small Spatula Saucepan (check the bowl sits in/on it) Measuring spoons – tbsp 1lb Loaf tin (Simple Kit) / Foil Tray	50g GF biscuits 100g GF Chocolate 40g Marshmallows 40g Raisins	65g *butter/dairy free block 2tbsp Golden syrup

Let's Bake.
Make sure your baking area is clean, pop on an apron, tie your hair back & wash your hands.

METHOD

Step 1	• Line a 1lb loaf tin with clingfilm or lightly grease the foil tray (you could use clingfilm instead). • Half fill the kettle & boil. It doesn't need to boil, just be hot – **Ask an adult for help.**
Step 2	• In a large metal or glass bowl, add your butter, chocolate and golden syrup. • **If you are using a measuring spoon, put it in a mug of hot water first so it warms & the syrup will slide off the spoon easily. Or weigh 30g of syrup into the bowl. It's the same.
Step 3	1) Your bowl needs to sit on the top of the saucepan, with the bottom resting in it - known as a Bain Marie (a water bath). The bottom of the bowl shouldn't touch the water. Make sure it's a good fit before adding the hot water into the pan. 2) **Ask an adult to help -** Place the saucepan on the hob, pour in 3-4cm of hot water from the kettle. Sit the bowl on top of the saucepan. 3) Gently melt the butter, chocolate & syrup together, stirring occasionally. 4) When melted, remove the bowl from the saucepan and let it cool for 5 minutes on the side.
Step 4	While the mixture is cooling, put the biscuits into a bowl and break them into small bite size pieces.
Step 5	• Add your raisins & bite sized biscuit pieces to the chocolate mix. • Stir until well combined. • Add the marshmallows & stir well again until everything is coated in chocolate.
Step 6	• Pour the mixture into the prepared tin/foil tray. • Scrape out the bowl, and press/push the mixture into the corners so it is almost level. • Place the foil tray onto a plate or baking tray to put it into the fridge. • Pop it into the fridge for 1-2 hours to set firm.
Step 7	• *After 1-2hrs, check to see it is firm to touch. Take it out of the tin, remove the clingfilm & place it on a chopping board.* • ***Ask an adult for help*** *to cut it with a sharp knife. Cut it into slices and then small squares. Keep it in a airtight box in the fridge.*
OPT.	*You could add various extras if you wanted. 2-3 tbsp of GF rice krispies or GF cornflakes, a few chopped glace cherries, mini eggs or Moo Free GF/DF mini eggs. Or drizzle it with melted white chocolate for special occasions.*

Gluten Free Little Cook Recipe – Vanilla Cookies

Equipment Required	Dry Ingredients (supplied)	Wet Ingredients (not supplied)
1 x large & small mixing bowl Spatula/Mixing Spoon/ Fork 1 tbsp (tablespoon) Baking tray/ *Greaseproof paper Rolling Pin / Weighing scales Cling film *cookie cutter	125g Gluten Free Plain Flour 62.5g Caster Sugar ¼ tsp Xanthan Gum Icing Sugar Icing Pen GF Sprinkles	1 egg (you only use half!) 1 tsp Vanilla Extract 62.5g Butter – Room Temp *If using dairy free 'butter'* *you must use a block butter* *– I used Flora Plant*

Tie your hair back, wash your hands & pop on an apron
Check you have a clean area for cooking.

METHOD

Step 1	Cream your butter & sugar together. In a large mixing bowl, add your butter. Squish it a bit with your spatula so that it softens more and is easier to mix together with the sugar. Add the sugar to your butter and mix well until all combined.
Step 2	Crack your egg into the smaller bowl. Check for any shell bits. Beat the yolk and white together in the bowl with the fork.
Step 3	Add **half** the egg and 1 tsp of vanilla extract You only need half of the egg. You can try to pour half into the butter mixture or use a tablespoon to scoop about 3 tbsp into the mixture. Mix well.
Step 4	Add your GF plain flour & Xanthan Gum. Mix together until a ball of dough is formed. Once your dough is in a ball, you need to wrap it in clingfilm and chill in the fridge for 20-30 minutes.
Step 5	Tidy up & get ready to roll!! Prepare your baking tray. Either use greaseproof paper or lightly oil your tray and sprinkle a little flour on top to stop your cookies sticking. • Lightly flour your work surface. Unwrap your dough and put it onto the flour • Pop the palm of your hand flat onto the flour and rub your floured palm over your rolling pin so that it doesn't stick to your dough when you are rolling it out. • As you roll out your dough – don't press to hard – you will need to lift the edges gently, turning the dough so that it doesn't stick. If it gets stuck or sticky, sprinkle a little flour under the dough, or re-flour your rolling pin. • Roll out gently until it is the thickness of a £1 coin.
Step 6	• Time to cut out your cookies by placing the cutter onto the dough and gently pressing down. • Lift out/up and put onto the prepared baking tray spacing them out evenly • Add eyes/features with the end of a teaspoon. • Chill your cookies again on the tray for 20m before cooking. **Pre-heat your oven to 160c**
Step 7	*Bake your cookies for 6 minutes. Turn the tray round & cook for a further 4-6m. Once they are beginning to colour/go golden brown at the edges, they are cooked. Cool on the tray for 5 minutes and transfer to a wire rack using a palette knife.*
Step 8	*Add the icing sugar to a small bowl. Add 1-2 tsp of warm water to the mixture. Mix well. Once your cookies are cold, decorate as you choose with icing and sprinkles.*

Gluten Free Little Cook Recipe - Flapjacks

Equipment Required	Dry Ingredients (supplied)	Wet Ingredients (not supplied)
x large saucepan patula/Mixing Spoon Grater Baking tray Greaseproof paper (opt) Weighing scales Adult supervision	125g Gluten Free Oats 50g Raisins 50g Light Brown Sugar 50g Chocolate chips Foil Tray or use a 1lb loaf tin	100g butter (dairy or plant) 40g Golden Syrup **Small grated Vegetable or Fruit Vegetable oil for greasing the tin

**Adding fruit or vegetables into our flapjacks will help our tummies and digestive systems which do an important job keeping us well.*
Why not try adding one of the following to the above recipe & let me know what you think is the best flavour.
*Select an item from box **1-3** below:*

1	2	3
A small grated apple, piece of Carrot, Parsnip or Sweet Potato	Small piece of fresh grated ginger, 1 tsp Cinnamon or Ground Ginger	Select one: Raisins, Chocolate Chips, Dried Coconut, Dried Pineapple, Dried Mango

Some flavour combinations below. What would you mix together?

Apple & cinnamon	Raisins & Carrots	Parsnip & Raisins	Mango & Coconut	Pineapple & Chocolate	Carrot & Fresh Ginger

Method

Step 1	Preheat the oven to 160c. Grease the silver tray / 1lb loaf tray. You might want to use greaseproof paper to line the 1lb tray so it comes out easily.
Step 2	In a large saucepan melt together the butter, sugar and golden syrup together.
Step 3	Remove from the heat, and cool for 5 minutes. If using, grate your chosen vegetable/fruit – maybe a small apple or half a carrot. **If it's very wet when grated, squeeze a bit of the juice out of it.**
Step 4	Add your oats & raisins into the melted butter mixture and stir well. Really get those arm muscles working!! When mixed well & all the oats are covered in the butter mixture, add your grated vegetable/fruit. Stir well until combined.
Step 5	Put the mixture into the silver tray / 1lb loaf tin. Press it down into the corners with your spatula & flatten it slightly. Not too much.
Step 6	Place the filled tray onto a baking sheet & put into the centre of the oven. Cook for 25-30 minutes until golden & firm to touch
Step 7	Remove from oven when cooked. Leave on the side to cool. Melt the chocolate in a microwaveable bowl in 10-15 second bursts until melted. Use a teaspoon to scoop up the melted chocolate and drizzle it over the flapjack when it is cold. Cut evenly and eat. *Remember that by adding fruit it will make your flapjack more moist than normal.* *For regular flapjacks exclude the fruit.*

Gluten Free Little Cook Recipe - GF PlayDoh

Equipment Required	Dry Ingredients
1 x large mixing bowl 1 x medium saucepan (bigger one if you double the mixture) Whisk Spatula American measuring cups Tablespoon Plastic gloves to knead in colour Baking paper	½ cup of rice flour ½ cup of cornstarch / cornflour ¼ cup of table salt 2 tablespoons cream of tartar 1 cup of water 1 tablespoon of oil – vegetable or coconut Gluten Free food safe colouring

Tie your hair back, wash your hands & pop on an apron.
Wipe down your kitchen cooking surface so it's clean and ready to go!

Method	
Step 1	• Add all your dry ingredients into a medium sized saucepan. • If you double up, use a bigger pan.
Step 2	• Mix your dry ingredients with a whisk
Step 3	• Add the water and oil to the dry ingredients. • Stir well
Step 4	• Cook over a medium heat • Continue to stir as it becomes thicker so it doesn't catch on the bottom of the pan • Scrape down the sides and across the bottom of the pan continuing to stir
Step 5	• Once thickened, remove from the heat • Stir so it comes into one big ball • Tip the ball onto some baking paper whilst it cools
Step 6	• As it cools and becomes easy to handle, cut the ball into half and into quarters • Add some GF food colouring to each quarter • Put on some plastic gloves & work the food colouring into each quarter • Squash and squeeze the food colouring so the playdoh has the colouring mixed evenly. Once it is mixed, it won't stain your hands or your child's!!
Step 7	• Store in an airtight container in a cool place. It should last a few weeks before you need to replace it. • Wrap it in clingfilm before placing in the container to keep it nice and soft
Step 8	To make it smell nice, you can add a drop of essential oil – but I'd do this after you tip it out of the pan – you could then knead it through the playdoh. Using coconut oil helps change the smell of the dough. Salt makes it less palatable if they decide to try to eat it! Super salty! *Original recipe by Katie at Wheat by the Wayside.*

Section 9

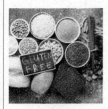

1 FIRST STEPS

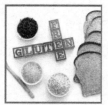

2 WHAT DOES GF MEAN?

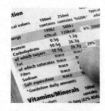

3 READING LABELS

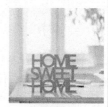

4 HOME LIFE & EATING OUT

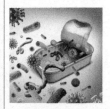

5 CROSS CONT- AMINATION

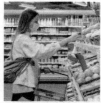

6 SHOPPING/ SNACKS/ TRIPS OUT

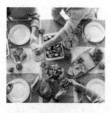

7 FOOD IDEAS

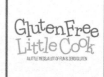

8 GFLC RECIPE FUN

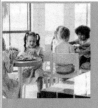

9 NURSERY & SCHOOL

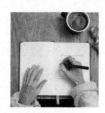

10 USEFUL INFO

Nursery & School

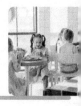

Initial Steps

I didn't have to put my gluten free coeliac child through nursery. She wasn't diagnosed until she was 9. That was hard enough but our school understood her needs.

As a trained nursery nurse, I've spent time in nurseries and schools over the past 20-30 years. Some things don't change!

They will still be making pasta shapes pictures, making foods with wheat flour, using play-doh (yes, gluten is in that too!) & sensory play with cornflour. Cornflour is fine by the way!

You need to get the importance of keeping your child safe and on a gluten free diet across.

My suggestion is that you put in in writing at all times. That way you have proof that you've advised them. Always ask for a written response from the nursery or school so you have a written timeline.

Nursery & School

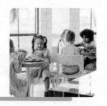

Initial Steps

Nurseries and schools like your child to be officially diagnosed nowadays. That's why it is important to get your child tested properly at the beginning.

- Have your child's dietitian write to the nursery or school
- Put your child's detailed requirements in writing stating about gluten free food needs.
- Give them a printout showing what is safe/what isn't - make it clear
- Ask for a written response within 7 days so they confirm they understand your child's needs.
- **Provide them with a *Coeliac UK School Pack* - download from their website**
- Ask that they arrange an appointment with their Senco so you can get a secure healthcare plan in place.
- Keep everything in a file so you have it to hand easily

Nursery & School

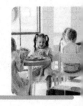

Initial Steps

Ask them to keep you informed if they are having a special celebration so you can provide safe gluten free alternatives.

For example:

- Flapjacks for health week
- Pancakes for Shrove Tuesday
- Cake sales - provide a GF cake for your child in a sealed plastic box labelled especially for them, stating gluten free.
- Birthday treats - it's birthday madness in the early years. All their peers celebrate by bring in treats. Make a treat box (name & label) to take in & be held by the teacher, fill it with tasty GF treats, then when a birthday occurs they can choose a safe substitute. Restock as required.
- Snacks - nurseries/schools often have biscuits as treats. Ensure they have a stock of GF biscuits too!
- Get a good level of communication going with their main teacher.

Nursery & School

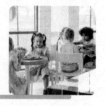

UK Guidance

England

- The Children's and Families Act 2014 came into force in September 2014, and states that all state funded schools in England, including academies and free schools in England **must make arrangements for supporting children with medical conditions**. The Act also places a duty on these schools to offer a free school lunch to all pupils in reception, year 1 and year 2.

Northern Ireland

- Free school meals are not universal but are available for some children depending on individual circumstances. Check to see if your child is entitled to free meals.

Scotland

- Since January 2015, the Scottish Government has provided free school meals for all children in primary 1 to 3 across Scotland.

Nursery & School

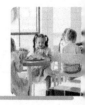

UK Guidance
Wales

- In Wales, all primary school children are entitled to a free school breakfast. Free school meals are not universal but are available for some children depending on individual circumstances.

Check what is available in your area.

If your child is entitled to a free school meal, they shouldn't be excluded because they have Coeliac Disease. They should make provision for them. There are no excuses. And it shouldn't be just salad, jacket potatoes and plain cooked chicken.

Your child should not be excluded from any activity regarding food. They should be able to provide a safe suitable alternative.

It isn't hard to do and to get it right.

Nursery & School

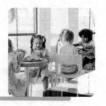

UK Guidance

Under section 100 of the **Children & Families Act 2014** , schools have a duty to support pupils at their school with medical conditions.

In schools, kitchen staff need to be able to easily identify those with specific dietary requirements. Practices to identify children with dietary needs could be as simple as:

- coloured wrist bands
- a photograph of the child alongside details of their allergy in the kitchen or serving area
- lanyards, badges or different coloured trays

Now some children don't like being identified - but it helps the staff. And it's important that the kitchen staff follow your wishes - staff stating "oh my friend has coeliac disease, she can eat normal pasta, just gives her a funny tummy" isn't what you want to hear.

It's important to make them understand early that your child can't eat gluten for their health.

Nursery & School

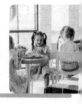

Governmental Acts

Do look at 'Supporting pupils at school with medical conditions' Dec 2015. It's a 29 page document and worth looking at to put your point across for back up if needed.

Look at **Annex A** - Model process for developing individual healthcare plans. *Screen shot on following page.*

- Pupils at school with medical conditions should be properly supported so that they have full access to education, including school trips and physical education
- Governing bodies must ensure that arrangements are in place in schools to support pupils at school with medical conditions
- Governing bodies should ensure that school leaders consult health and social care professionals, pupils and parents to ensure that the needs of children with medical conditions are properly understood and effectively supported

Nursery & School

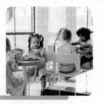

'SUPPORTING PUPILS AT SCHOOL WITH MEDICAL CONDITIONS'
DEC 2015.

Annex A: Model process for developing individual healthcare plans

Parent or healthcare professional informs school that child has been newly diagnosed, or is due to attend new school, or is due to return to school after a long-term absence, or that needs have changed

⇩

Headteacher or senior member of school staff to whom this has been delegated, co-ordinates meeting to discuss child's medical support needs; and identifies member of school staff who will provide support to pupil

⇩

Meeting to discuss and agree on need for IHCP to include key school staff, child, parent, relevant healthcare professional and other medical/health clinician as appropriate (or to consider written evidence provided by them)

⇩

Develop IHCP in partnership - agree who leads on writing it. Input from healthcare professional must be provided

⇩

School staff training needs identified

⇩

Healthcare professional commissions/delivers training and staff signed-off as competent – review date agreed

⇩

IHCP implemented and circulated to all relevant staff

⇩

IHCP reviewed annually or when condition changes. Parent or healthcare professional to initiate

GlutenFree
Little Cook

Notes

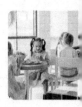

Make notes here - what to tell your child's nursery or school
How will they distinguish your child at lunch time?
How will they keep her safe?
Tell them to call you if in doubt.

Notes

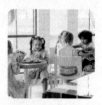

Section 10

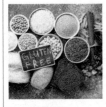

1 FIRST STEPS

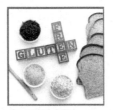

2 WHAT DOES GF MEAN?

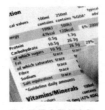

3 READING LABELS

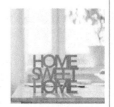

4 HOME LIFE & EATING OUT

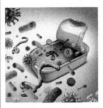

5 CROSS CONT-AMINATION

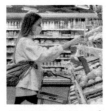

6 SHOPPING/ SNACKS/ TRIPS OUT

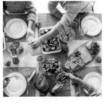

7 FOOD IDEAS

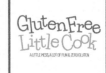

8 GFLC RECIPE FUN

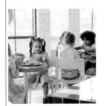

9 NURSERY & SCHOOL

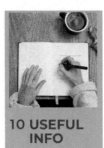

10 USEFUL INFO

Useful Info

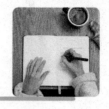

Extra help & support

Coeliac UK

They've a wealth of information, various apps, Facebook group, website and Instagram.

They have an awareness campaign each year, highlighting the disease. I highly recommend you joining it to support them, the research into the disease & much more.

A yearly membership includes the apps, with either a digital guide or a hard copy via post.

Websites

When googling, do be sure to look for UK based sites.

- The UK spelling of the disease is 'Coeliac'. The USA version is 'Celiac'.
- If you see Coeliac written as the USA version, you are best to head out of that website and go to a UK based one.
- Do your own research

Useful Info

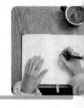

Extra help & support

The 20ppm

I've not mentioned it as it isn't on any label. Anything under 20 parts per million (20ppm) is acceptable to someone with Coeliac Disease according to the law in the UK and that product can be labelled as gluten free.

But it's not on any label for a reference. Therefore if an item is labelled gluten free, then those levels are below 20ppm.

America / Australia variations

Australia has a slightly different outlook on gluten free vs the UK. They don't recommend eating any GF oats in your diet at all.

They have a lower limit of 5ppm.

Useful Info

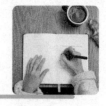

Facebook Groups
Facebook
There are lots of gluten free groups on Facebook. You'll need to find the group that is right for you.

Search for Coeliac, Coeliac Disease, Gluten Free & they'll come up. I suggest you look for groups that are UK based to save any confusion.

Group suggestions:
- Gluten Free UK
- Children with Coeliac Disease
- Coeliac Children UK
- Coeliacs in the UK
- Coeliac Disease Support Group
- Coeliac Sanctuary
- Coeliac Disease for Beginners*

Note: Everyone has their own advice & it isn't always uptodate if they're diagnosed several years ago. **Do your research on Coeliac UK.**

Useful Info

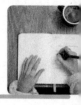

Groups

Key bloggers & Instagram accounts I find value in:

- Gluten Free Little Cook (hey, that's me!!)
- Becky Excell - The Gluten Free Blogger
- The Loopy Whisk - Katarina Cermelj
- Coeliac Dietitian - Cristian Costas - Instagram
- Kids Coeliac Dietitian - Natalie Yerlett (Dietitian)- Instagram
- Life on a Rice Cake
- Bakeritablog - superb gf sourdough starter & bread guides

On Instagram
On Facebook
On Both

Notes

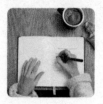

What do you need to remember?

Thank you

I do hope that this book helps you when you start out on your gluten free, coeliac disease journey with your child.

In 2018, I didn't know what I was going to do. How it was best to help my child. I didn't know anyone who had the disease. That could help her.

But I, like you, had to learn fast to get her back to health. Several years down the line, she is much better. She grew in height over 2" in the first year.

There's much to learn about Coeliac Disease, it's not just about cutting out the gluten. Hopefully this helps you to to start & feel more secure in what you need to do.

They say there is a book in everyone. Here's mine. Wishing you well & the very best for the future. If you have questions, contact me.

Nicky

GlutenFree
Little Cook

Printed in Great Britain
by Amazon